Dr lauson meletis

Things you don't know about Achalasia

How to live a fulfilling life irrespective of the challenges of a live long disease

First edition

This book was professionally typeset on Reedsy
Find out more at reedsy.com

Contents

1. INTRODUCTION TO ACHALASIA...1

Detailed explanation of what Achalasia is: 1

Types of Achalasia 1

Historical context of Achalasia...1

2. CAUSES AND RISK FACTORS 9

Achalasia Causes 9

Neurological factors or causes of Achalasia....................................9

What is the neurological cause of achalasia? 9

Genetic predisposition affecting Achalasia 9

3. SYMPTOMS AND DIAGNOSIS 13

Symptoms of Achalasia 13

Diagnosis for Achalasia...13

4. MEDICAL TREATMENT...17

Suitable treatments for Achalasia..17

Botox injection 17

5. SURGICAL OPTIONS 20

Peroral endoscopic myotomy 20

Heller myotomy...20

Fundoplication surgery 20

6. LIFESTYLE AND DIETARY CONSIDERATIONS 24

Dietary modifications and eating strategy 24

Lifestyle adjustments...24

7. LIVING WITH ACHALASIA...27

Strategies for maintaining a fulfilling life despite the challenges. ...27

A patient story who had Achalasia 27

8. CONCLUSION 46

Can Achalasia kill ? 46

Support groups and helpful resources for Achalasia patients..........46

    1.

        1.

        2.

        3.

    2.

        1.

        2.

        3.

        4.

    3.

        1.

      2.

    4.

        1.

        2.

    5.

        1.

        2.

        3.

    6.

        1.

2.

7.

1.

2.

8.

1.

1

INTRODUCTION TO ACHALASIA

Detailed explanation of what Achalasia is:

Achalasia otherwise called cardio spasm is an

uncommon problem making it hard for food

and fluid to pass into the stomach.

Achalasia can typically be made do with

negligibly obtrusive (endoscopic) treatment

or medical procedure.

Also, Achalasia can be explained as the

absence of esophageal peristalsis and

impaired relaxation of the lower esophageal

sphincter (LES) in response to swallowing

are hallmarks of achalasia, a primary

esophageal motility disorder. The LES is

hypertensive in around half of patients. At

the gastroesophageal junction (GEJ), these

abnormalities result in a functional

obstruction.

It is a deadly disease which not well taken

care of will certainly affect the heart and

cause more damage than expected.

Types of Achalasia

1.Classic Achalasia or type 1 Achalasia : Classic achalasia is another name for type 1 achalasia. Because the muscles in this type of esophagus barely contract, food falls only because of gravity.

2.Type 2 Achalasia: With this kind, the throat muscles scarcely contract, so food drops down in light of gravity alone. The esophagus becomes compressed in Type 2 achalasia as pressure builds up. This is the most widely recognized kind of achalasia and it frequently causes more extreme side effects than type I.

3.Spactic Achalasia or type 3 Achalasia:

Spastic achalasia, also known as type III achalasia, has a mean IRP that is higher than the upper limit of normal, there is no normal peristalsis, and at least 20% of swallows

have preserved fragments of distal

peristalsis or premature (spastic)

contractions.

Historical context of Achalasia

Sir Thomas Willis, an English physician and

one of the Royal Society's founders, first

described the condition that is now known as

achalasia in 1672 and treated it with a

dilation using a sea sponge attached to a

whale bone.

Johann Freiherr von Mikulicz-Radecki, a

German, Polish, and Austrian physician,

identified the condition as cardiospasm in 1881 and believed it to be a functional rather than mechanical issue.

Ernest Heller was the first person to successfully perform an esophagomyotomy, which is now known as the Heller myotomy in his name. In 1929, two doctors named Hurt and Rake discovered that the issue was caused by the LES not relaxing. They named the infection achalasia, meaning powerlessness to unwind.

F.C. Lendram used the term achalasia rather than cardiospasm to support Hurt and Rake's findings in 1937. Difficult to say who truly changed the name between the last two

sections) In 1937, the doctor F.C. Lendram

confirmed the finishes of Harmed and Rake
in 1929, sending the use of the term

achalasia over cardiospasm.

Rudolph Nissen, a German physician

who was a student of Ferdinand Sauerbruch,

performs the first fundoplomy in 1955,

which is now referred to as the Nissen

fundoplication. He eventually published the

results of two cases in a 1956 issue of Swiss

Medical Weekly. In 1962, Dor reports the first

anterior partial fundoplication, which acts as

a solution to the intense post-surgery GERD

and the risk of stomach acid inhalation that

is associated with Heller myotomy.

The first posterior partial fundoplication

was reported by the doctor Toupet in 1963. In

England, the first laproscopic Heller's was

performed in 1991 by the doctor Shimi and

his colleagues.

In 1994, Paricha et al. introduces Botox as

a means of reducing pressure in the LES.In

2008, H. Inoue in Tokyo, Japan, developed

the most recent method of surgically treating

achalasia: the per-oral endoscopic myotomy.

This method is currently regarded as

experimental in many nations including The

United   States.

2

CAUSES AND RISK FACTORS

Achalasia Causes

One is connected with degeneration of the

nerve cells situated between the layers of

esophageal muscles. The esophagus can

move food toward and into the stomach

thanks to these nerve cells. A correlation

between achalasia and parasitic or viral

infections has been suggested by some

studies.

It has been consequently proven over the

years that external factors like population

affect achalasia and it has Been observed that

the more the population get higher the more

the chances of having achalasia In such

environment gets higher and it is mainly

caused by the inflammation of the

oesophageal myenteric plexus which elicits

an auto immune response.

Neurological factors or causes of Achalasia

What is the neurological cause of achalasia?

The exact cause of achalasia is not known.

Some clinical researchers suspect that the

condition may be caused by the degeneration

of a group of nerves located in the chest

(Auerbach's plexus). It is believed that there

may be a rare, inherited form of achalasia,

but this is not yet well understood at this

time.Patients with achalasia have autonomic

nerve dysfunction in the vagal nerve outside

the esophagus.

Genetic predisposition affecting Achalasia

Achalasia must be considered for

differential diagnosis in children with

positive family history of achalasia even in

the absence of typical clinical

manifestations. An autosomal recessive

mode of inheritance is probable.
For example few weeks ago

A 5-month old boy was hospitalized for

cough and mild respiratory distress. Because

of positive history of achalasia in his mother,

achalasia was detected in esophgagography.
Pneumatic dilation through endoscopy was

successful.

NOTE: Achalasia can happen at any age but it

mostly frequently occurs in age 30-60

3

SYMPTOMS AND DIAGNOSIS

Symptoms of Achalasia

Symptoms of alchalasia include:

Regurgitation (food coming back up),

weight loss, chest pain, and cough are

some of the symptoms of achalasia. Other

symptoms include difficulty swallowing and

food "sticking" in the esophagus. Medicines

mean to make it simpler for the food to pass

from the throat into the stomach by relaxing

the muscles engaged with this interaction.

Dysphagia: The medical term for difficulty swallowing is dysphagia. Dysphagia is a condition that can be painful. Occasionally, swallowing is difficult. Occasionally having trouble swallowing, like when you eat too quickly or don't chew your food well enough, is usually nothing to worry about. Difficulty swallowing can have causes that aren't due to underlying disease. Examples include large bites of food, inadequate chewing, dry mouth, pills or food that's too hot. Swallowing is also difficult when talking, laughing or lying down.

Regurgitation: Regurgitation happens when a mixture of gastric juices, and sometimes undigested food, rises back up.

Causes include: smoking, pregnancy ,eating disorders,lying down immediately after eating , heart burn

Chest pain: Chest pain can be referred to as a dull ache in the chest, a crushing or burning sensation, a sharp stabbing pain, and pain that spreads to the neck or shoulder are all symptoms of this condition.

Normal CAUSES

Chest agony can have makes that aren't expected hidden infection. Models incorporate truly difficult work, power lifting, injury to the chest or gulping a huge piece of food.

Diagnosis for Achalasia

Manometry is quite often used to affirm the

determination of achalasia. The test

ordinarily uncovers three irregularities in

individuals with achalasia: low (peristaltic)

contractions in the lower esophagus,

inability of the LES to relax after swallowing,

and elevated LES pressure at rest.
We have several types of manometry and

that depends on the situation of such patient

or   the   type   of   Achalasia   he/she   has.

4

MEDICAL TREATMENT

Suitable treatments for Achalasia

P robably the most common treatment for

achalasia is balloon dilation. Most patients

(65% to 80%) report a critical improvement

of gulping after the strategy. However, the

improvement may only last a short time;

achalasia symptoms may recur over time and

necessitate additional treatment.

Botox injection

The injection of botulinum toxin into a

muscle temporarily paralyzes that muscle for

months to over a year. Botulinum toxin is

mostly used to treat achalasia in

gastroenterology. The lower esophageal

sphincter muscle is injected with botulinum

toxin.

Before eating, your doctor may

recommend muscle relaxants like

nitroglycerin (Nitrostat) or nifedipine

(Procardia) or calcium channel brokers.

These medications have severe adverse

effects and little effect on treatment. In most

cases, medications are only considered if you

are not a candidate for surgery or pneumatic

dilation,   and   Botox   has   not   helped.

5

SURGICAL OPTIONS

Peroral endoscopic myotomy

Peroral endoscopic myotomy is a procedure

to treat swallowing disorders caused by

muscle problems such as spasms in the

esophagus. POEM uses an endoscope — a

narrow flexible tube with a camera — that is

inserted through the mouth (peroral) to cut

muscles in the esophagus (a myotomy).

Cutting the muscles loosens them and

prevents them from tightening and

interfering with swallowing.

POEM is not considered a surgery, since no

incision is made through the skin. It is a less

invasive alternative to Heller myotomy — a

similar procedure that uses small incisions to

reach the esophagus instead of access

through the mouth. Endoscopic procedures

often mean less pain and a faster recovery

than open surgical procedures.

Heller myotomy

Heller myotomy is a surgical procedure in

which the muscles of the cardia are cut,

allowing food and liquids to pass to the

stomach. It is used to treat achalasia, a

disorder in which the lower esophageal

sphincter fails to relax properly, making it

difficult for food and liquids to reach the

stomach.

Fundoplication surgery

Fundoplication surgery wraps the upper

stomach around the lower esophagus. It

reduces the amount of acid that enters the

esophagus from the stomach. This procedure

can: Eliminate gastroesophageal reflux

disease (GERD) symptoms that are not

relieved   by   medication.

6

LIFESTYLE AND DIETARY CONSIDERATIONS

Dietary modifications and eating strategy

Adopt a soft textured diet. For more severe

cases, a pureed or liquid diet may be needed.

Incorporate soft cooked, mashed or pureed

foods; soups, smoothies and crock-pot

meals (tender meats and vegetables).

Smoothies and protein shakes are especially

helpful when appetite or intake is low.
Take small bites, chew food thoroughly and

limit stressful distractions at meal times. Do

not go to bed immediately after a meal. Allow

about three hours after eating before laying

down to prevent regurgitation and

heartburn.

Lifestyle adjustments

Changing your diet.

Choose foods that pass more easily down

the esophagus like liquids or soft foods. Eat

problem foods like grisly meats, dry foods, or

raw vegetables and fruits with care. Eat

several small volume liquid or semi-liquid

meals throughout the day and avoid large

meals.

Best foods to eat are fish meat cereals bread

and   lastly   fruit   and   vegetables.

7

LIVING WITH ACHALASIA

Strategies for maintaining a fulfilling life despite the challenges.

T here is no "one size fits all" approach to

achalasia because individual experiences can

vary greatly. When it comes to food, for

instance, some people have bad experiences

with certain kinds of food, but this may not

be the case for others. Even brands of food

that are similar to one another can have

different effects. Additionally, problem foods

frequently have inconsistent effects on an

individual, causing regurgitation or reflux on

one day but not on another.

Achalasia patients who have only recently

been diagnosed with the condition or even

those whose condition has worsened over

time despite a number of medical

interventions may have different experiences

than those who have received successful

treatment.

Over the course of a number of years,

Achalasia Action has amassed a wealth of

useful information and tips. This includes

information about medications, nutrition,

how to deal with painful spasms, and

potentially harmful foods. These clues might

should be changed and deciphere by

individual requirements, like seriousness of

side effects, and whether you have been

treated with a surgery.

For successful management of chronic

conditions, behavioral and lifestyle

adjustments are required. Most of the time,

patients manage their chronic diseases in

their daily lives; However, for information

exchange, decision-making, and motivation,

their interaction with healthcare providers is

crucial. Persistently sick patients need to

deal with their everyday living under various

monetary and social imperatives, and their

related side effects can confound the most

normal exercises of day to day living. As per a

review did by Clark et al, three separate

classes of exercises should be addressed to

effectively self-manage a constant condition.

To begin, individuals with chronic

conditions require sufficient knowledge of

their condition and its treatment in order to

make well-informed decisions. Second, in

order to manage their condition, they must

engage in activities by altering their lifestyle,

including their diet.. Thirdly, they need to

learn how to work, keep a healthy family,

and build social connections in order to

maintain adequate psychosocial functioning.

The goal of these self-management

activities is to make chronic conditions less

of a burden on daily life.

Living with a chronic condition,

especially a rare one like achalasia, is

difficult. When someone suffers from a

disease that is easily visible or well-known,

the general public frequently shows

compassion and understanding; However,

people and those with whom they come into

contact face a variety of difficulties when

they live with a disease that is either obscure

or uncommon. Factors that facilitate

adaptation and adjustment to a chronic

condition that lasts a long time include

knowledge, coping strategies, and problem-

solving abilities. People are better able to

deal with their anxiety and uncertainty when

they have a better understanding of their

condition, whereas people who lack

knowledge feel powerless.

A patient story who had Achalasia

Kim's Story – Achalasia

''My name is Kim and this is my story

after recently being diagnosed with

Achalasia. My hope through writing this, is

that it helps someone else who is suffering

with the same thing or is waiting for a

diagnosis and has similar symptoms.

My story starts in June 2016. I'd been

living in Spain for 6 years, working as an

English teacher, loving both my job and the

Spanish life style. I was always busy with

teaching and lesson planning, but also found

time to go to Zumba classes twice a week and

go out with friends at the weekends. One day,

a completely normal day at home, I had

lunch and then was suddenly sick after

eating. I didn´t think much of it and

continued with my normal routine. This

being sick went on for 3 days but I finally

gave in when it got to the point that I was

being sick after sipping water and went to

A&E in Spain. There I was told I had

gastroenteritis and I was admitted to

hospital for 3 days as I was severely

dehydrated and the doctors seemed worried

that I was living on my own. After 3 days on a

drip in hospital, I was discharged and told to

keep an eye on my symptoms and if things

flared up, to go back to A&E. Over the next 3

months, I was in A&E 10 times due to

vomiting, dizziness and fainting, only to be

told each time that it was gastroenteritis and

it would clear up on its own.

In September 2016, I felt my symptoms

weren´t clearing up on their own, so I saw my

Spanish GP. She gave me a prescription for

paracetamol and ibuprofen for 6 months and

to go back in 6 months' time if my symptoms

weren't any better. Things seemed to get a

bit better, I was only having a bad day of not

being able to eat anything at all once a

fortnight, so I got on with my life. At this

point I was still teaching every day and going

to Zumba classes when I could. December

2016 was when things really started to get

worse. I was now being sick nearly every day,

so I went back to the Spanish GP. She told me

I was stressed and she could prescribe me

antidepressants. I kindly refused and got on

with things on my own. However, from

December 2016 to March 2017, the sickness

got worse, resulting in various hospital trips,

and now I was being sick 3 times a day, every

time I ate. Again, I went back to my GP, who

this time said it might be a food intolerance

so we went down the route of lactose and

gluten testing, which came back negative. I

was told I had to figure out on my own

exactly what I was allergic to. I knew it wasn

't an allergy, as everything was making me

sick. It didn´t matter what I ate, or how

much, I would be sick after eating or having a

drink. At this point I had to drastically reduce

my hours at work, as I was being sick, feeling

dizzy, and was so tired all the time. I also

stopped going to Zumba classes. Eventually

in August 2017, I'd had enough with Spanish

doctors and being on my own, so I came back

to the UK and saw a doctor here.

The first step in returning to the UK was

getting through to doctors here. The first

doctor I saw at my local doctor's surgery

again told me it was all in my head and that I

was imagining these symptoms, or it could

be stress-related. However, I wasn't

stressed, just frustrated that no-one believed

me! I gave up with the GP. Move on a few

weeks down the line and I saw another GP at

the same surgery. The day I saw him, I'd

been in bed for 4 days previously, having

been sick every day, suffering with

abdominal pain, feeling very dizzy, fainting,

and sleeping so much as I was so tired. This

GP believed me that something was wrong as

I could barely walk from reception into his

room for the consultation. He made some

calls and sent me straight to hospital for

further tests and investigations. I was

admitted for 2 and half weeks. During this

time, I had an endoscopy, colonoscopy, a CT

scan and a 24-hour heart monitor, due to

fainting episodes while I was on the ward.

After this hospital stay, the second step,

since giving up work, was to sort out some

financial support for myself. I was first put

on Job Seekers allowance, but about 2 weeks

in to the process, I saw a very helpful woman

who was a benefits advisor. She understood

straightaway that I couldn't hold down a job,

or even be looking for a job and attending

interviews. She said my health had to come

first. All she needed to move me onto ESA

(currently Universal Credit) was a sicknote

from a doctor. The nice GP who I'd seen,

kindly obliged, and I was moved onto ESA,

meaning I didn't have to worry financially

and could focus on looking after myself

instead of looking for a job.

After being discharged from hospital, I

was now under gastroenterology and had a

list of pending tests. This was the start of

many, many tests and appointments with the

gastroenterologist, each to no avail and only

to be told they would do more tests. All in all,

from December 2017 to October 2018, I had 2

gastric emptying studies (after not being

able to complete the first one due to

throwing up), another endoscopy (during the

first one, no photos were taken, so I had to

go through the whole thing again), 2 MRI

scans, 2 CT scans, and 3 ultrasounds. Yes, the

doctors were very thorough, and every 3

months I´d have a follow-up appointment

with the gastroenterologist, only to be told

that nothing was showing up on the tests. I

was pleased when they kept saying it wasn´t

anything serious and nothing to worry about,

but I was still worried as I knew something

was wrong but doctors didn´t know what.

Even my GP called me his favourite

mystery patient and was running out of tests

to do. At this point I was desperate as I was

suffering with abdominal pain, feeling very

tired all the time, and being sick after eating

and drinking. I was able to tolerate breakfast

without any problems but after that, no

matter what I ate during the rest of the day, I

was sick. I´d been prescribed medication to

help with the acid reflux and heartburn,

which seemed to be under control, but I was

losing weight due to not being able to eat

properly. When I was discharged from

hospital, I was prescribed Fortisip drinks but

all I really wanted was to be able to eat a meal

without being sick afterwards.

In October 2018, I went to a hospital in

Leeds to have a manometry (swallow

function test) which wasn´t the nicest of

tests, but it turned out to be the test that led

to my diagnosis. Later this month I saw the

gastroenterologist who told me I had

Achalasia as the muscles in my oesophagus

don´t work properly. After nearly 2 years of

hospital visits, tests, going round and round

in circles, being told it was all in my head, I

finally had a diagnosis and a name for my

disorder. This was a huge relief. Now I am

trying to find a way to manage this disorder.

I am currently taking antibiotics, before

returning to the consultant in 3 months to

see what other options there are. I have a

feeling it will be a case of managing the

symptoms on my own and researching the

disorder the best I can, with little support

from the doctors. It´s a wait and see game´´.

Well I hope you gained some knowledge from

Kim's   story   and   experience.

8

CONCLUSION

Can Achalasia kill ?

People don't typically die because of achalasia.

Although it tends to be a lifelong condition, with

symptom management, you can avoid the most

serious complications of achalasia, such as

aspiration, choking and malnutrition. People

with achalasia tend to have a higher risk of

developing esophageal cancer.

However, There's no cure for achalasia. Once the

esophagus is paralyzed, the muscle cannot work

properly again. But symptoms can usually be

managed with endoscopy, minimally invasive

therapy or surgery.

Also, if achalasia is untreated for a prolonged

period of time, the esophagus may become

enlarged and eventually stop working.

Researchers have noted that patients with

untreated achalasia have 16 times the chance of

developing a form of cancer known as

esophageal squamous cell carcinoma (ESCC).

Support groups and helpful resources for Achalasia patients

There are several health tips which have been

stated earlier that's are good goldmine as

well as great tips and knowledge for

Achalasia patients.

Futhermore, there are also non

governmental organizations or groups such

as Achalasia Awareness organization(AAO)

etc that organize varieties of programmes for

those affected with achalasia which will

make them not to feel bad or think and make

them live a fulfilled life.

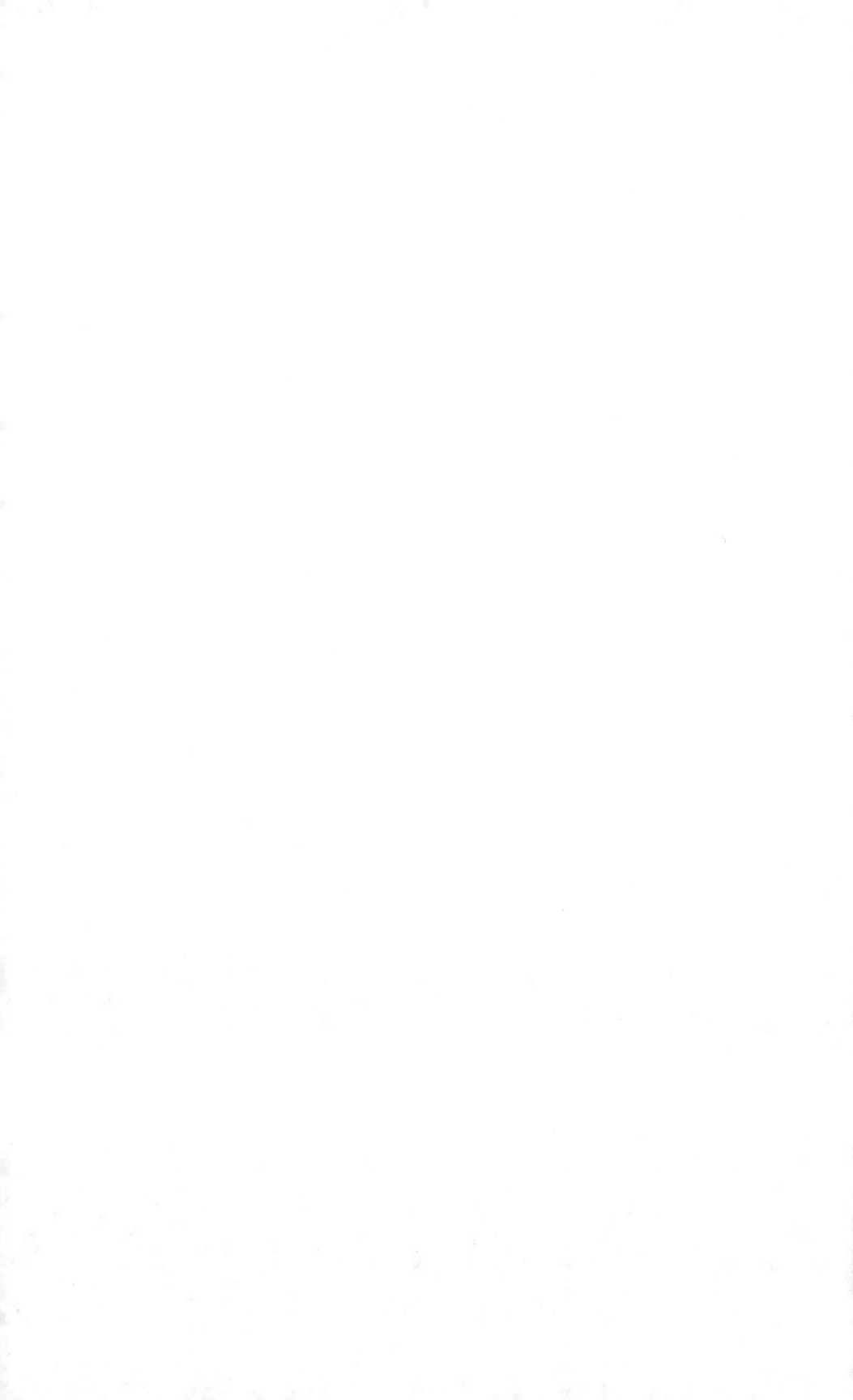

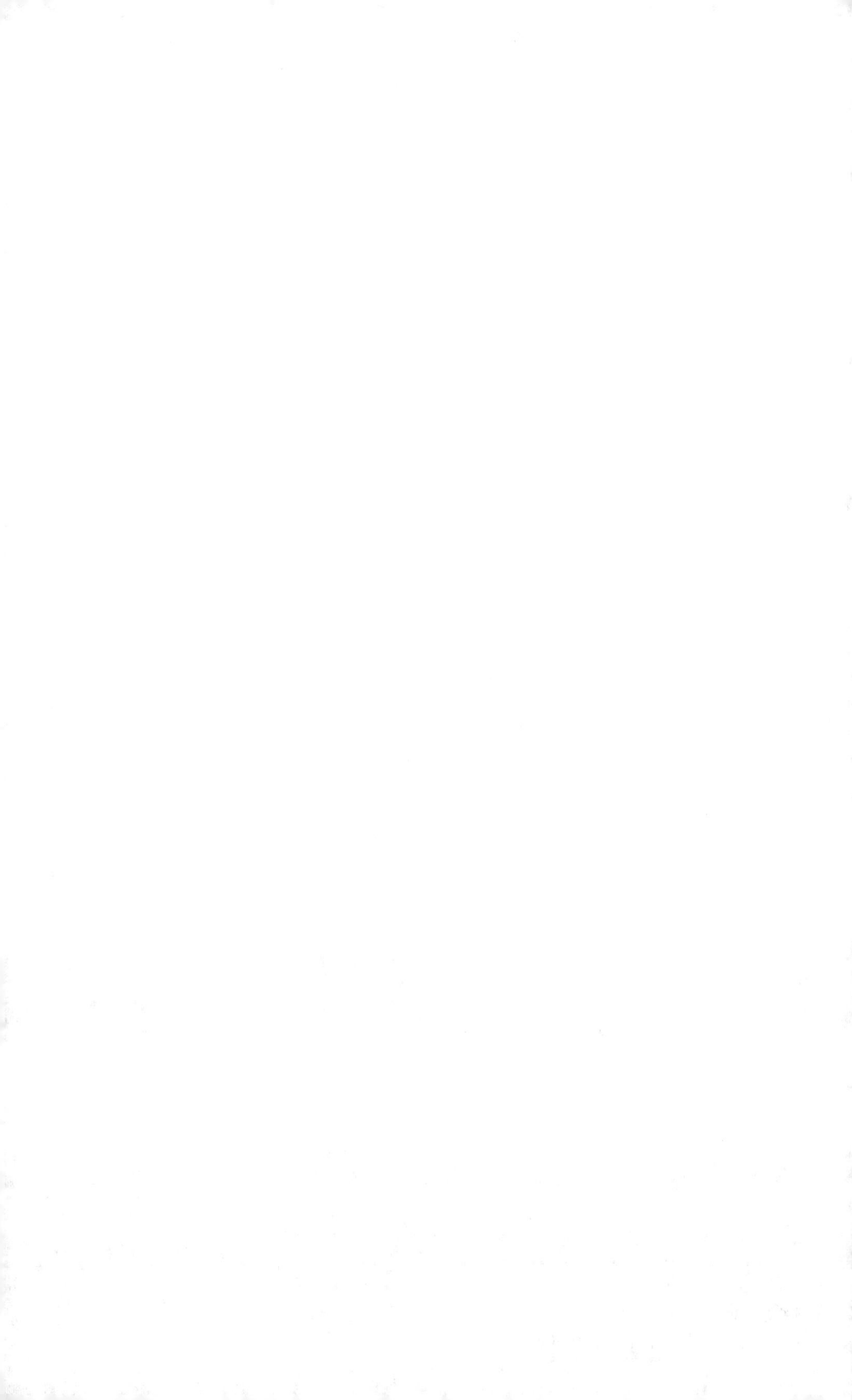

www.ingramcontent.com/pod-product-compliance
Lightning Source LLC
Chambersburg PA
CBHW062259290526
45794CB00006B/2613